Animal Healthcare Training

Case Study
Animal Healthcare Training

Nepal's animal health improvement training programme

John Young, Karen Stoufer, Narayan Ojha, Henk Peter Dijkema

Edited by Sarah Jones

Intermediate Technology Publications 1994

Intermediate Technology Publications,
103/105 Southampton Row,
London WC1B 4HH, UK

© Intermediate Technology Publications 1994

ISBN 1 85339 245 6

Printed by Russell Press, Nottingham, England

Cover photo: © IT/John Young

In the same series
Village Animal Healthcare: A community-based approach to livestock development in Kenya

CONTENTS

Figures and Tables vi
Preface vii
Acknowledgements ix
Acronyms x

Introduction
    Background 1
    Setting 2
    Livestock disease and animal health services 4

Animal health improvement training programme 8
    The farm and veterinary clinic 9
    The training course – selection and content 10
    The beginners course 12
    Training resources 13
    The medicine kit 17
    The refresher course 19
    AHITP follow-up role 20
    Refresher course survey 21

Field visits 22
    Introduction 22
    Palpa District 24
    VAHWs in Baugha Pokhara Thok 31
    South Lalitpur 33
    VAHWs in South Lalitpur 38

Conclusions 41

Appendices 46
    Appendix 1: Diseases treated by the VAHWs 46
    Appendix 2: Beginners' course contents 48
    Appendix 3: Refresher course contents 49
    Appendix 4: The AHITP recommended medicine kit 50

FIGURES

Figure 1	Map of Nepal showing mountain, mid-hill and Terai zones
Figure 2	Location of VAHWs
Figure 3	RDC structure
Figure 4	Illustration from trainee textbooks
Figure 5	Illustration from trainee textbooks
Figure 6	Illustration from liverfluke flash cards
Figure 7	Map of Baugha Pokhara Thok
Figure 8	Livestock calendar in Baugha Pokhara Thok
Figure 9	Beanograms of problems in Baugha Pokhara Thok
Figure 10	Map of Pyutar
Figure 11	Beanograms of problems in Pyutar

TABLES

Table 1	Distribution of land, cultivated land and human and livestock population by agroclimatic zones in Nepal
Table 2	Village animal health workers trained per district
Table 3	List of questions taught to trainees
Table 4	List of skills needed to give an injection

PREFACE

This book describes one of the longest-running village animal healthcare projects that I know about. It started in the early 1980s shortly after the idea of modifying the Chinese Bare-Foot Doctor approach for use in animal healthcare emerged among community-based development agencies. It was among the first projects to try this approach. That the project is still running, and generating increasing interest among the farmers and government staff of Nepal, is testament to its validity. Since then many other projects have followed a similar approach.

The problems, successes and lessons of this first project have been widely incorporated in others. The issues raised by this work in Nepal – access to medicines, the scope of the training, integration into government services and sustainability – are common to all. The Animal Health Improvement Project has been dealing with these issues longer than most, and the story should be essential reading for those thinking of embarking on a similar project.

This story has been compiled from many sources. Much came from the results of a comprehensive evaluation of the project undertaken in November 1991. This has been suplemented by a paper on the project presented at an international conference by Karen Stoufer and Narayan Ojha in 1992, and an update on the project written by Henk Peter Dijkema in 1993.

This publication is part of a series of case studies published by Intermediate Technology on this topic. An earlier title – *Village Animal Healthcare* by Grandin, Thampy and Young, IT Publications 1991 – has proved popular. This new title will be a useful addition to knowledge and experience on the subject.

John Young
Nairobi, 1993

ACKNOWLEDGEMENTS

The evaluation team would like to thank all the farmers and village animal health workers in Ikudol, Pyutar, Asrang and Baugha Pokhara Thok for patiently answering all their questions. Also Jagath Barjgain and other staff of the CDHP Lalitpur and Lila Jhirel and other staff from CHP Tansen who organized and participated in the two field trips; Jhaman Singh Dorlami who allowed the team to stay in his house in Baugha Pokhara Thok; Alison Craven of the INF, Tom Arens of World Neighbors, Luminath Adhikari of the CDHP, Gerrit ten Velde of the Lutheran World Service and Babu Ram Pathak of Action Aid Nepal, Dr K.R.Panday the Director of the Department of Livestock Services, Dr Hans Dhal of the Livestock Breeding Project, and staff of the Department of Livestock Services in Kathmandu, Lalitpur and Tansen, who all made time available for interviews. And finally, Keith J. Fisher and other staff of the RDC Pokhara for providing transport and computing facilities.

This book could not have been produced without the support of all the staff of AHITP throughout its prolonged gestation, and the efforts of Sarah Jones who pulled all the different documents together.

LIST OF ACRONYMS AND DEFINITIONS

AHITP	Animal Health Improvement Training Programme
CBS	Central Bureau of Statistics
CHDP	Community Health and Development Project
CHP	Community Health Project
FAO	Food and Agriculture Organization
GTZ	German Agency for Technical Development
IFAD	International Fund for Agricultural Development
INF	International Nepal Fellowship
ITDG	Intermediate Technology Development Group
JT(s)	Junior Technician(s)
JTA(s)	Junior Technical Assistant(s)
RDC	Rural Development Centre
UMN	United Mission to Nepal
VAHW(s)	Village Animal Health Worker(s)
VDC(s)	Village Development Committee(s) an administrative area, previously called the Panchayat
Dharmi Jhankri	A type of traditional healer
Pradhan Panch	Chairman of the former Panchayat
Ropani	Measure of land area: 20 Ropani = 1 Hectare, 8 = 1 Acre
Murrah	Kind of sheep

INTRODUCTION

Background
The United Mission to Nepal was founded in March, 1954 to send Christian medical missionaries into Nepal. Hospitals were set up as well as centres for rural healthcare. Once in Nepal, the UMN rapidly expanded into other areas of development work such as education, agriculture, and engineering. Based on reports from farmers in the UMN's community health project areas of the need for training in animal health in the villages, the Animal Health Improvement Programme (AHIP) was conceived in 1980 with the aim of training project staff and farmers in simple animal healthcare techniques.

Since 1981, formal training courses for Village Animal Health Workers have been conducted by a staff of both expatriate and Nepali animal husbandry specialists, veterinarians, livestock educators and animal health technicians at the Mission's farm in Pokhara. While both training methods and course content have continued to evolve over the years in response to trainee requests, the growth of development work in Nepal and programme experience, no formal evaluation of the programme is now known as the Animal Health Improvement Training Programme (AHITP) had been undertaken.

In 1991, anticipating change in the government's livestock policy with the arrival of democracy in Nepal, AHITP staff decided to conduct their own evaluation with the assistance of a veterinarian from Intermediate Technology and a local agriculturalist. The goals of the evaluation were to determine whether there was a continuing need for improved animal health services, and to assess the effectiveness of the programme in terms of the quality of the training courses, support to trained village animal health workers (VAHWs), their continued efficiency, and the benefits to the farmers. A broader aim of the review was to help AHITP define a strategy for the future within the expected restructuring of the government's Department of Livestock Services (Ministry of Agriculture).

The evaluation was based on information already held within AHITP, on material from other sources, some new information from projects, a survey of VAHWs attending a refresher course, and on two field visits to Lalitpur and Palpa Districts. The areas were chosen for their relative accessibility and, as they had previously been designated by AHIP as 'saturation' sites, both had many VAHWs who had been working for a number of years and good information was available from their projects (the Community Development and Health Project (CDHP), Lalitpur, and the Community Health Project (CHP), Palpa).

The findings of that evaluation are presented here with additional information on the training programme taken from a paper given by Dr Karen Stoufer and Dr Narayan Ohja. This opening section includes the setting and a discussion of the need for improved livestock healthcare in Nepal. The second section describes the AHITP, its existing structure, the course content, the materials it produces and the medicine kit it provides. It also includes the conclusions of the refresher student interviews. The third section is an account of the two field trips to Lalitpur and Palpa, the methods of data collection, and some discussion of the findings. The final section outlines the general conclusions and the recommendations of the evaluation.

Setting

Nepal is a small land-locked nation of 18 million people, with an area of approximately 56,000 square miles (about 147,000 square kilometres) of which 35 per cent is high mountains. The Great Himalayas, including the highest peaks in the world, form the northern border with Tibet (the People's Republic of China) and a narrow strip of flat, fertile sub-tropical farmland forms the southern border with India. Nepal is primarily an agricultural country. Over 90 per cent of people work on farms, and agricultural products produce about 60 per cent of the country's Gross Domestic Product and half of its exports. Over half of the farms are less than half a hectare in

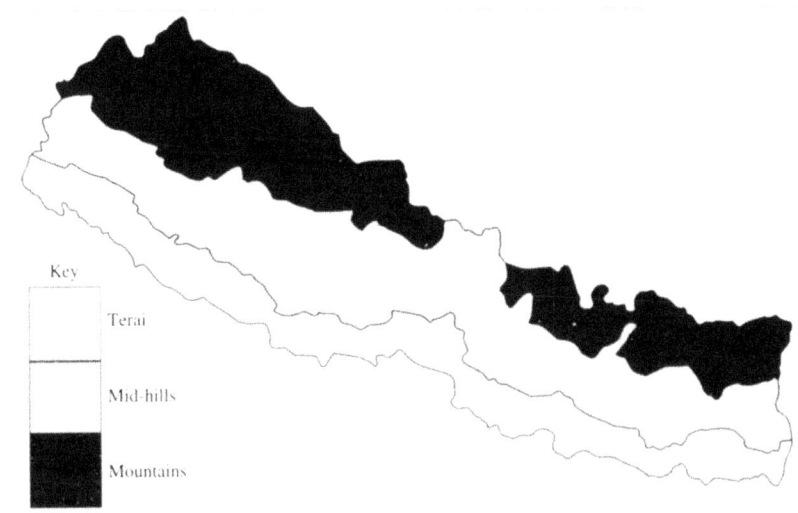

Figure 1: Map of Nepal showing mountain, mid-hill and Terai zones

total area, most are fragmented into several small pieces, and production is primarily at subsistence level. Nepal has more livestock per hectare of cultivated land than anywhere else in the world (4 cattle and 2.5 small ruminants – *FAO Production Yearbook 1986*), and livestock numbers are increasing. They form an essential component of most agricultural systems, providing draught power and manure for fuel or fertilizer. They provide meat, milk, and eggs for food or sale for cash, fibre, hides and skins, as well as fulfilling important social and religious functions. Livestock are estimated to contribute about 15 per cent of the country's Gross Domestic Product, and are an important source of cash revenue for farmers in the hill and mountain regions where they contribute about 20 per cent of household income. The steeply terraced hills and river valleys of the mid-hill region are intensively cultivated, and support the largest part of the population. This region, which has more than half of the national livestock population, is where the field sites of Lalitpur and Baugha Pokhara Thok (Palpa District) are located.

Table 1: *The distribution of land, cultivated land and human and livestock populations by agroclimatic zones in Nepal*

Zone	Total area %	Cultivated area %	Human population %	Livestock Population			
				Cows & buffalo %	Sheep & goats %	Pigs %	Poultry %
Terai	23	58	44	11	20	12	12
Mid-hills	42	37	47	54	55	60	62
Mountains	35	5	9	35	25	28	26
Total (000s)	147,151 (sq. km)	2,287,496 (ha)	15,022,839	9124	5667	442	9187

Source: IFAD Special Programming Mission to Nepal 1989
CBS Comparative Study of Ecological Belts 1981-82

Livestock disease and animal health services

A 1991 GTZ funded evaluation of the impact of disease on livestock productivity in six districts in Nepal estimated that parasitic diseases, mainly liverfluke, intestinal worms and lice and ticks accounted for 34 per cent of total disease losses, worth about Rs. 25 million (£350,000) annually. A further 34 per cent was lost due to foot and mouth disease. Other major diseases were tick-borne diseases, haemorrhagic septicaemia (HS) and brucellosis. The total annual loss from disease in the six districts is estimated at Rs. 50 million (£700,000).

In 1991 there were 156 veterinarians in Nepal. Of these, 82 provide services to farmers from 75 District Livestock Development Offices, usually in the District headquarters. They are assisted by 1520 Junior Technicians (JTs) and Junior Technical Assistants (JTAs) working from the Livestock Development Offices and 729 Livestock Service Centres in the rural areas. The service is free of charge to farmers who bring animals to the centres, but there are severe budgetary constraints for drugs and vaccines, and centres often run out. Because of these difficulties and the lack of an adequate road system in rural areas it has been estimated that these services only reach about three to five per cent of livestock owners in the country (Livestock Master Plan – 1991).

There are no specific data on the livestock health status of the two field-site areas. However, through discussions with farmers, VAHWs, JTAs and veterinarians some information was obtained. In South Lalitpur, the commonest diseases are liverfluke, internal and external parasites, foot and mouth disease, haemorrhagic septicaemia and anthrax. Progeny histories showed that loss from disease is a major problem especially for young animals. The District Veterinary Hospital in Lalitpur is in Patan, five kilometres from the centre of Kathmandu, and about forty kilometres from Ikudol, Pyutar and Asrang, the three villages surveyed. There are seventeen livestock sub-centres in the District, with the nearest at Battedanda, about four hours walk from the villages. There has been no JTA at Battedanda for the last five months, and the sub-centre often has little medicine.

Access to veterinary services is similarly limited at the field site of Baugha Pokhara Thok near Tansen, the closest government veterinary facility being the veterinary hospital in Tansen itself, about two hours walk from the village. In addition, however, there are eleven veterinary sub-centres in the district.

While livestock disease proved to be a central concern of farmers in both Lalitpur and Tansen, other problems such as the lack of forage and the shortage of water and labour were also felt to impose severe constraints on livestock production. With the increase in population over the last ten years, more land is being cultivated and less is available for grazing. Deforestation has also reduced the available forage for grazing animals, and to protect community forestry people have voluntarily restricted grazing and keep their animals stall-fed, bringing fodder to them. At the same time as the population has expanded, households have become smaller with people tending to live in nuclear rather than extended families and with children more likely to attend school. As a result, many households have a shortage of labour which directly affects their capacity to care for their livestock. Livestock health and production in the country must now be seen in the context of a changed social and agricultural climate, where livestock disease represents only one element.

Since the Animal Health Improvement Programme began in 1981, the programme has trained 364 VAHWs in twenty districts in the mid-hills of Nepal. The number trained and their location are shown in Figure 2 and in Table 2.

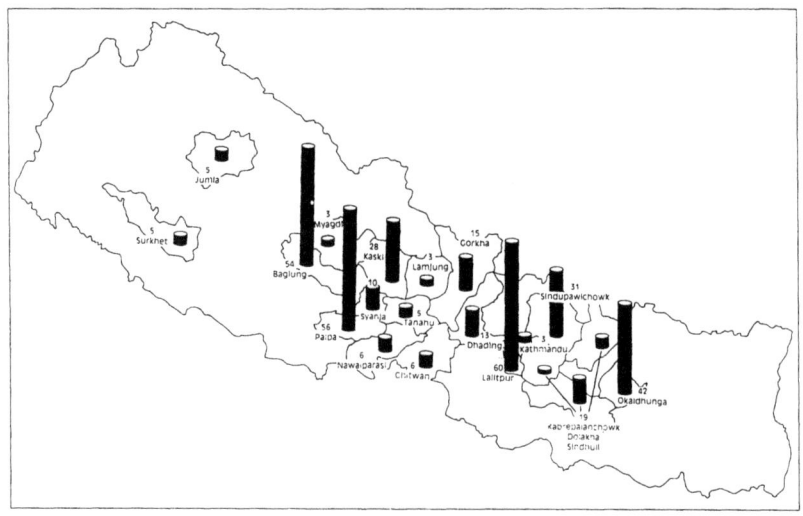

Figure 2: Location of VAHWs

Of the information available on VAHWs trained by AHITP, 74 per cent are still working at least one year after training. Of VAHWs trained up to three years ago 75 per cent are still working, as are 72 per cent who were trained more than five years ago. There appears to be no significant difference in the 'drop-out' rate between women and men, but evidence from follow-up visits is that some women are prevented from working by their husbands.

Information on the work done by the VAHWs after training is incomplete until 1989, but available records indicate that they have been vaccinating animals against haemorrhagic septicaemia and

Table 2: Village Animal Health Workers trained per district (1991)

Mid-Western Region		Central Region	
Jumla	5	Chitwan	6
Surkhet	5	Dhading	13
Total	10	Kathmandu	3
		Lalitpur	60
Western Region		Kabrepalanchowk	2
		Dolakha	5
Baglung	54	Sindhuli	12
Myagdi	3	Sindupawlchowk	31
Palpa	56	Total	132
Syanja	10		
Kaski	28	**Eastern Region**	
Lamjung	3		
Tanahu	5	Okaldhunga	42
Nawalparasi	6		
Gorkha	15		
Total	180	**TOTAL NEPAL**	**364**

other diseases, and treating a wide range of diseases, including internal parasites (worms and liverfluke), mange and other skin diseases, intestinal problems, infections, injuries and obstetrical problems. They also perform a number of simple routine procedures including castrations and horn cutting. (A table of VAHW treatments derived from AHITP follow-up visit reports in several project sites is given in Appendix 1.)

THE ANIMAL HEALTH IMPROVEMENT TRAINING PROGRAMME

In 1978, in response to the requests for animal healthcare training for farmers, a UMN veterinarian who was running the farm at Gandaki Boarding School designed two experimental training courses. The first was a short (three-day) course held for farmers in different villages close to Tansen in Palpa. This proved to be largely unsuccessful as the farmers were unwilling to allow the trainers or trainees to handle their animals. The need to organize practical hands-on training resulted in a two-week course for project staff held on the GBS farm, Lamachaur, in Pokhara District. The farm was found to be an ideal setting; not only did it have its own animals, but the animals of neighbouring farmers were being brought to the farm for treatment. The Animal Health Improvement Project was born of the success of this trial course.

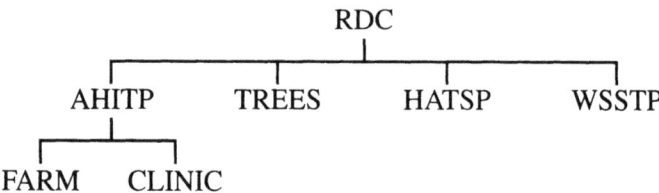

Figure 3: RDC structure

In mid 1981, the Rural Development Centre (RDC) of UMN was established as a consultancy service to provide technical expertise to UMN community development projects in Lalitpur, Palpa and Gorkha in animal husbandry and health, forestry, water supplies and horticulture. Once established, the RDC took over the GBS farm as part of its operations. The AHITP forms part of RDC (see Fig. 3) providing training rather than consultancy expertise in the areas of animal husbandry and health. Since 1987, RDC's three other programmes, Forestry (Trees), Drinking Water Systems (WSSTP) and Horticulture and Agronomy (HATSP), have evolved into training rather than consultancy services.

The farm and veterinary clinic

The farm, covering just over three hectares, is primarily a livestock farm with 40 per cent of the land used for fodder and fruit trees, 35 per cent for fodder grass and fodder grain crops, and 25 per cent for buildings and pathways. Most of the fodder produced is for the farm's own livestock, which includes seventeen breeding goats and their offspring, five male goats, seven breeding rabbits and offspring, one milking buffalo and calf, two oxen, two fattening pigs and about twenty chickens. The buildings consist of offices, animal buildings, a classroom and two dormitories for the male and female trainees, a kitchen, and the clinic.

Although an expensive operation, the farm serves a number of functions. As a training centre for VAHWs it is able to demonstrate housing, feeding and general animal care techniques with healthy animals on the farm itself and the farm animal health clinic can provide cases to be used for teaching purposes and for practical treatment experience. Small-scale livestock trials (e.g. the monitoring of productivity of livestock) are conducted, thus providing some research background to support choices in course content.

The farm's fodder production, including short term crops, maize and oats, fodder trees and grass and the preservation of excess fodder such as silage and hay, the stall feeding of animals, and the results of a comprehensive preventative treatment of livestock against parasites are all examples of the farm's activities. Other small-scale trials have included, live fencing, cropping under trees, grass yields, green manuring, silage making, hay making, and a goat cross-breeding trial which monitors the growth rates of offspring.

Local farmers have been bringing animals to the farm for treatment for over twenty years, but the veterinary clinic was only officially established at AHIP's commencement in 1981. Animals brought to the centre are treated for the cost of the medicines used plus 25 per cent to cover administrative costs and losses. While the clinic staff will attend animals at home for a small fee, farmers are encouraged to bring animals to the farm, when possible, so that clinical material is available for trainees during the courses. The clinic keeps records in a day book of all the animals treated. From these records, it appears that the range of cases seen at the clinic (listed in Appendix 1) closely matches those cases seen by VAHWs after training, making it a particularly useful teaching resource.

The clinic, initially run by the expatriate veterinary staff, who trained local assistants, is now run by one full-time and one part-time clinician. While neither clinician is a veterinarian both have had extensive VAHW training.

In addition to the farm and clinic staff, AHITP in 1991 employed five people to organize, develop and run the training courses. They include two expatriates, a veterinarian and an animal husbandry specialist, and three Nepali livestock trainers two of whom have agricultural degrees, and one a recently qualified Junior Technical Assistant. Of the five, two – the veterinarian and the JTA – are women.

The training course – selection and content

AHITP offers two village animal health worker courses. The first is a beginners' course to train selected farmers to become VAHWs in their communities, and the second is a refresher course for actively working VAHWs to review the material of the first course and expand and improve their treatment skills and animal husbandry practices. Usually the trainees will return for the second course one to two years after the first, occasionally later.

All trainees are sponsored by an organization involved in community development work in their area. The sponsor agrees not only to pay the fee for the training but also to provide on-going support for the trainee in the field after he/she returns. Some sponsors are community health and development programmes of the United Mission to Nepal and some are government programmes, but most are other private NGOs (non-government organizations usually with ties to international development agencies such as CARE, Save the Children, Lutheran World Service, World Neighbors, Action Aid, International Nepal Fellowship).

AHITP advises the sponsors on selection criteria based on its experience of successes and failures. AHITP recommends that candidates be selected on five criteria. First, they should be experienced farmers who have not only raised animals before coming to the course, but also own the animals so that when they return they can implement disease prevention programmes that serve as a demonstration to their neighbours. Secondly, candidates should be at least twenty-five years of age. The age criterion was suggested not only in line with the need for experienced farmers but also because many young people now leave their villages to go to cities for jobs or more education. AHITP's goal is to train someone committed to staying in his/her village and providing a long term service. Marriage can also be an important stabilizing factor.

The third related criterion is that any candidate should not have completed the tenth grade (school-leaving certificate level). People who have completed the tenth grade tend to leave for more education and are less content with the village-level work of the course. Some notable exceptions to this have been school teachers who teach in the local village school and do their VAHW work before and after classes. The ability to read and write simple Nepali is considered a necessity for proper use of medicines and record keeping. However, this does not necessarily mean a person must have attended school; some very successful trainees have never attended school at all.

The last but perhaps the most important criterion is that candidates be selected by the community from which they come. In order for VAHWs to work successfully, their community needs to be supportive and expecting to use, and pay for, their services.

Both the beginners' and refresher courses last two weeks and include eleven full days of instruction. They are usually held from November to March when farmers are free to leave their fields for a short time. The trainees sleep in the dormitories on the farm and meals are also provided there. Classes are held both outdoors and in a large classroom upstairs over the dormitory. The ideal class size is 15 but in practice varies from 13-20. Trainees are frequently divided into smaller groups of 4-5 to work closely with one trainer.

The beginners' course

The course begins with a full day on how to examine an animal brought for treatment. This incorporates a standardized format of eleven questions to ask every owner in every case, an examination of the animal from a distance and an orderly method of examining the animal up close, starting at the head and working towards the tail (see Table 3).

Table 3: List of questions taught to trainees

1. What is the problem? or Why have you come?
2. When did the problem start?
3. What part of the animal seems to be the problem?
4. How old is the animal?
5. How are your other animals?
6. Does the animal eat and drink? What?
7. Does it ruminate? (for ruminants only)
8. How are the stools and urine?
9. Is she pregnant? (for females only)
10. Does she give milk? Is production affected?
11. What other treatments/medications have you already carried out/given?

Once the trainees know how to approach a case all diseases can be taught according to the same format. This framework serves VAHWs well in the village as they attempt to recognize both familiar and unfamiliar diseases. They know that certain answers to the questions, a certain overall appearance and certain specific findings from close examination always suggest a specific disease condition.

Emphasis is given to the most common diseases they will see in the village and on preventative measures such as routine de-worming and vaccinations (a detailed outline of course content is given in Appendix 2). Record keeping is also taught as a method of continuing self-education.

The course is designed to be 'hands on' and practical with very limited lecture presentation. Outdoor sessions are held using the farm-owned animals for practice in restraint, injection, and medicine administration techniques. Clinic cases are all handled by trainees using the standard question and examination format with assistance provided in recognizing and treating diseases. Classroom sessions include demonstrations, laboratory exercises, slide shows, videos, filmstrips, discussions, puppet shows and short dramas.

At the end of the course an examination is given. Practical skills have to be demonstrated and students are interviewed individually about disease recognition and treatment protocols. Since most students have only limited literacy, no written exam is given. Demonstration of skills and verbal interviews take longer but are more representative of what the trainee can actually perform upon return to his/her village.

Following the examination there is a goal-setting session where the trainers assist the trainees in setting realistic goals for themselves that can then be discussed at the follow-up meetings. Goal setting might include questions such as: how many animals do you think you will treat for liverfluke disease? How many will you give medicine to as a part of a preventative de-worming programme? After which, an official certificate-giving graduation is held to emphasize the trainees' importance in their role as village animal health workers.

Training resources
All training materials and methodologies are designed to offer maximum support to VAHWs once they return to their villages. As follow up and on-going support to VAHWs is a key component of the AHITP, every effort is made to provide the necessary resources and

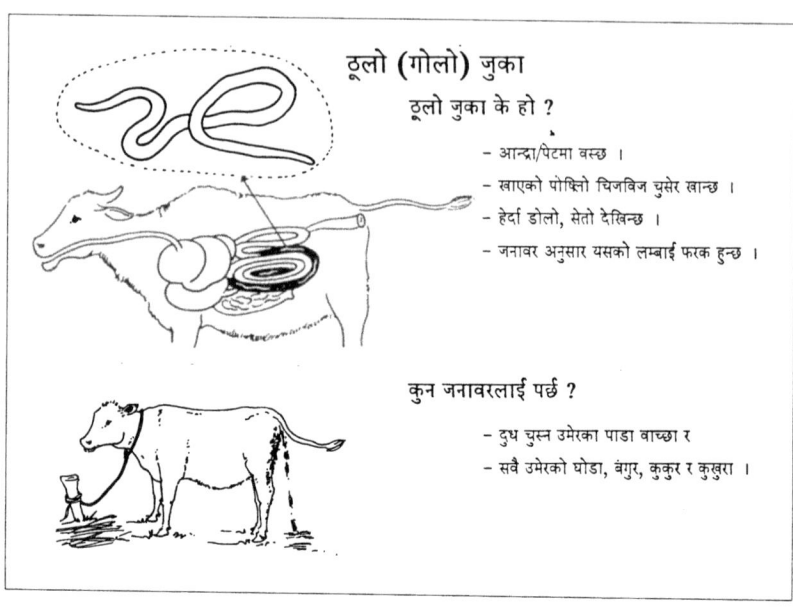

Figure 4: Illustration from trainee textbooks

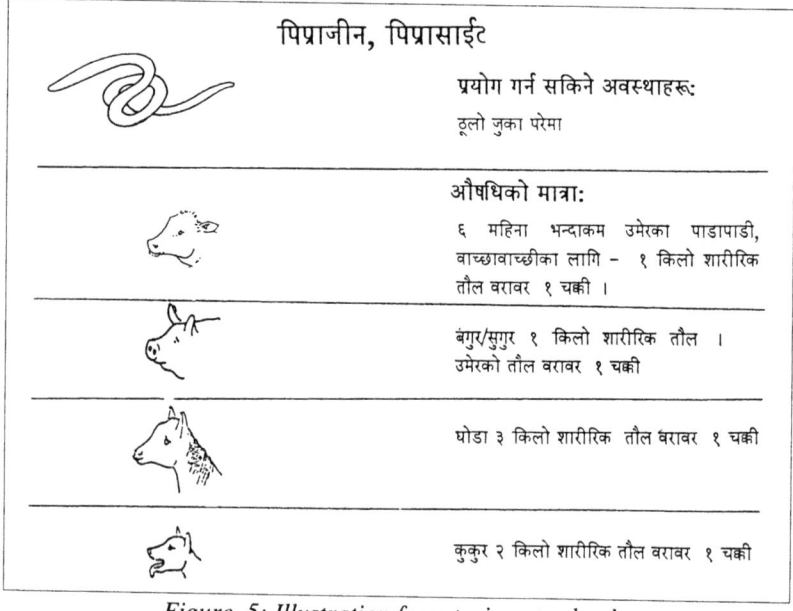

Figure 5: Illustration from trainee textbooks

experience it is felt they will need. Appropriate textbooks (see Figures 4 and 5) and audio-visual aids are used and later given to the trainees, field trips are organized, trainees are encouraged to give oral presentations on assigned topics using songs or dance to emphasize or illustrate a point, and they are also given the opportunity of talking to, and questioning an experienced VAHW.

Trainees are provided with a basic textbook and a medicine book which have simple text with many line drawings to illustrate the main points covered in class. Symbols are used to help the student find the appropriate section quickly and access material so that it can be used as a reference text at home after the course.

A combination of slide series, film strips, overhead projector transparencies, flannel board figures, flip charts and cardboard flash cards are used to illustrate discussions.

The flash cards, one on the work of the VAHW and liverfluke (see Figure 6), and one on detecting when female livestock are in heat, are designed for the trainee to be able to use in his or her own village as teaching material. A simple Nepali text is given with each picture.

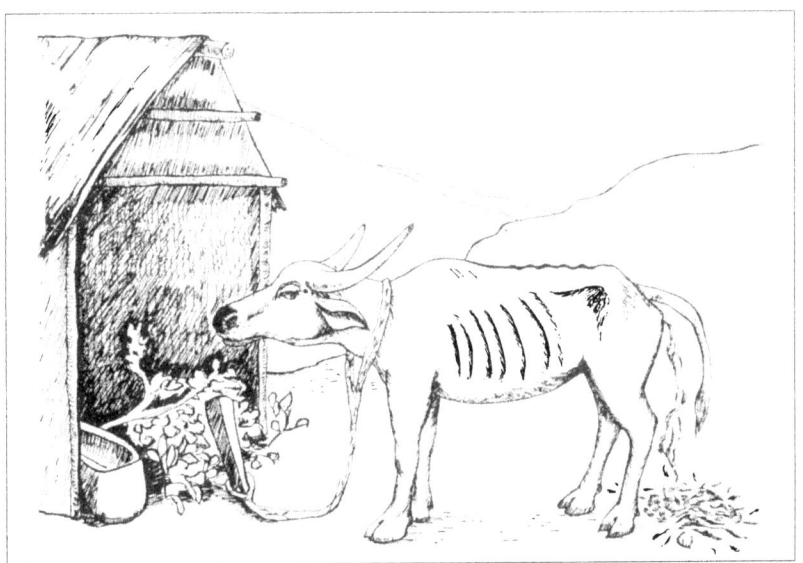

Figure 6: Illustration from liverfluke flash cards

Additional visual aids are used, such as: animal puppets, large cardboard and wood models of thermometers and a life size pelvis with a model calf to practise dystocia handling (difficult births).

Built into the second week of initial training is a question-and-answer session with the trainees and an experienced VAHW to 'tell it like it is'. Also, an AHITP-produced video of VAHWs working and being interviewed is shown to all trainees. As a further resource the clinic technicians also participate in the training, and discuss case handling with the trainees.

Table 4: List of skills needed to give an injection

1. Read the Arabic numerals on a syringe (Nepal has its own numerals and Devanagri script alphabet. Syringes and thermometers are only available with Western numerals so the trainees must learn to read the numbers).
2. Understand the meaning of the lines and intervals between the numbered lines on a syringe.
3. Put a needle on and off a syringe safely and without contamination.
4. Learn to put water into a vial and draw medicine out by appropriately using a measured amount of air and an 'in and out' technique.
5. Shake a vial to completely dissolve all medicine.
6. Remove air bubbles from a syringe of medication before administering an injection.
7. Measure the volume of medicine after mixing.
8. Mathematically split a dose (i.e. from a 40 unit bottle of medicine calculate how many ml will yield 10 units).
9. Clean and disinfect a syringe and needle before and after use.

All lesson plans are designed to be a simple step-by-step acquiring of knowledge and skills. An example of this is the lesson on how to prepare an injection. Every student is issued a syringe, needle, liquid disinfectant for cold sterilization of syringe and needle, glasses of water, paper and pen, and a vial of powdered medicine.

(Expired penicillin is supplied to AHITP in large quantities.) The trainer first performs the steps. Then a student trainee is asked to demonstrate a second time in front of the class. Next the trainees perform the skill themselves with several trainers present to assist and advise. This kind of skill training is just one approach used. Often a session will start with the trainer asking questions about trainees' experiences with a certain skill or subject. This usually leads to group discussions or activities where the trainer acts as a facilitator rather than an expert technician.

The component skills taught are illustrated on flip charts (poster size), demonstrated (down to the detail of actually boiling water in front of the class on a kerosene stove) and practised by each trainee in small groups.

A second class with a similarly prepared list of steps would follow on how to administer an injection to a particular animal. The first practice would be to administer an injection to a cardboard box. The second practice would be to administer an injection to a farm-owned goat and a farm-owned ox or water buffalo, and after that, to the village animal which comes for treatment.

In general terms of resources and methodologies, there exists little difference between the beginner and refresher course. The refresher course has the added resource of the trainees' experience.

The medicine kit

Of all the resources provided to trainees, the medicine kit is felt to be the most valuable. The programme recommends that all supporting projects provide an initial supply of medicines to each trainee. When this supply runs out, it is hoped that the trainees themselves will be able to restock with the fees they collect from the sale of the first issue medicines. Until 1992, to help projects accomplish this, AHITP offered two alternatives.

The first was that AHITP would provide a list of recommended medicines for a medicine kit and suggest reasonable quantities that should be provided. The project members would then buy the medicines themselves, following the AHITP guidelines.

The second, and now only, alternative was that the project staff would purchase a ready-made medicine kit in a lockable tin suitcase already prepared by the AHITP staff according to its own guidelines. When AHITP prepares the kit, all medicines included are exactly as taught in the course and are properly labelled with names, amounts and expiration dates in Nepali. For these reasons, it was decided that the latter alternative should be mandatory for all students.

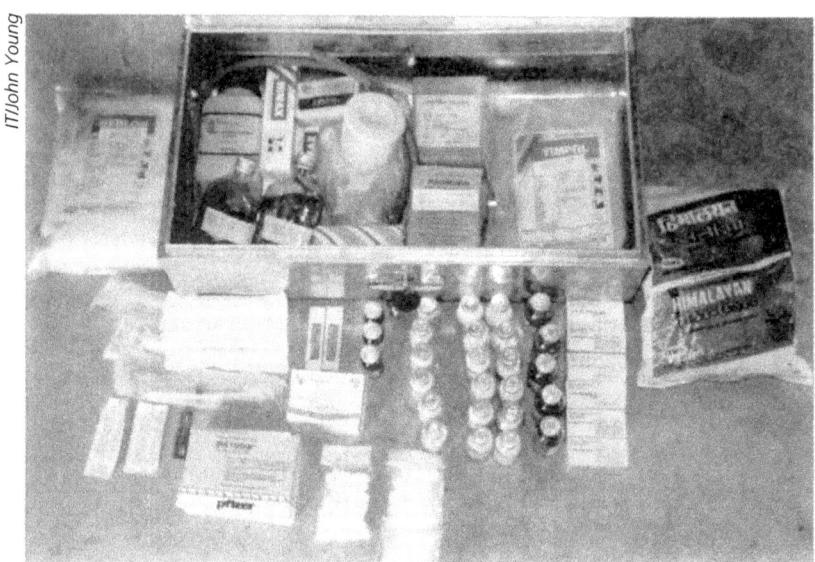

Medicine kit

A set of medicines has been prepared for the refresher course trainees including new medicines not covered in the beginner course. The refresher medicine kit was introduced in 1991.

The kits are designed with enough medicine so that the VAHW will not run out too soon, or have medicines left over after the expiration date. They include antibiotics, bloat medicine, diarrhoea medicines, de-wormers, external parasiticidal medicines, wound treatment medicines, needles and syringes, vitamin B, poisonous plant antidotes, uterine boluses, eye ointment, soap, cotton, goat stomach tube, and plastic for prepackaging medicines for sale in single dose quantities (the full contents of the medical kit are given in Appendix 4). AHITP charges Rs.2,500 (£35) for its kit, the cost of the medicines plus a 20 per cent handling fee.

The refresher course

The first three days of the refresher course are spent reviewing material from the beginner course, including a practical exam with staff and farm-owned animals role-playing to simulate real-life situations. Doing this in the first few days helps staff assess how much review is necessary, and for whom, and allows time for individual revision to be organized.

The subsequent eight days of instruction cover a range of topics, some of which are new to the trainees while others, i.e. the use of antibiotics, are a development and further analysis of subjects previously included in the beginners' course. A substantial part of the course is livestock husbandry and management, and related topics such as nutrition, stall feeding, hay making and the use of fodder trees. A full list of topics is given in Appendix 3.

In addition, the refresher trainees visit local farmers with improved breeds to learn the possible benefits of investing in purebreeds and their crosses as opposed to local breeds and also to see a variety of types of housing and management systems in operation. Visits to a poultry farm and a pig farm are organized for trainees to gain more experience with these species.

A new and popular element in the refresher course has been the addition of a trainee-run vaccine clinic in a nearby village. Not only does it provide a service to the community and injection practice for the students, but it shows the students how easily it can be done by them in their own villages.

Very important to refresher trainees is the opportunity to exchange experiences among themselves. This offers an occasion for the sort of problem-sharing lacking in their everyday practice. Classes are designed to build on this experience whenever possible.

AHITP follow-up role

Regular, consistent follow-up of VAHWs is seen as an important part of AHITP's work. AHITP staff personally aim to visit every trainee at his/her home within approximately six months of the training. They are accompanied by the sponsoring project's staff member responsible for the on-going support of the VAHW. Ideally, a project staff member will visit the trainees promptly after training to help get them started and then on a regular basis (such as 3-4 times a year) to help solve problems. AHITP now offers a course for project staff on how to conduct good quality follow-up for its VAHW trainees.

The AHITP follow-up visit usually includes meeting the trainee's family, seeing his/her own livestock and farmland, conducting a community meeting with the trainee, and holding a 2-3 hour review of the trainee's records, medicine supply and technical knowledge. The trainee has an opportunity to ask questions and present problems. Whenever possible the AHITP staff accompany the VAHW to see cases in the village.

When community meetings take place they usually include a discussion and survey of the main livestock-related problems in the area, such as feed, water, and diseases. Presentations are made on liverfluke prevention and treatment, on the VAHW and how farmers can best use his/her services followed by a general discussion of how certain local disease problems can be prevented or treated. The one-on-one review with the trainee ideally includes reading the case record book and discussing how each case was handled, difficulties encountered and the thoroughness of the recording itself. Medicine in the medicine kit is checked for proper labelling, expiration dates and the trainee's knowledge about its proper use. The trainee also demonstrates examination procedure and preparing an injection properly. If a trainee has forgotten certain lessons these are reviewed and if not, new topics or diseases he/she has encountered are taught. Finally the trainees are asked for suggestions on how the training course could be improved in the coming year based on their experiences during and after the course.

Refresher course survey
As part of the evaluation, trainees from Baglung District attending a refresher course were interviewed about their initial training, and their opinions of the teaching methods.

The trainees ranked liverfluke, the care of sick animals, advising farmers, restraint and the treatment of fleas and lice as the most useful topics on the beginners' course. Major infectious diseases were ranked low. Most (12 out of 15) felt the course should have been longer, some wanting more time to absorb the information which was presented, while others wanted more information. Their expectations for the refresher course were to learn about more diseases, especially red water which is a common problem in their home area (Baglung). Interestingly in a ranking exercise of topics likely to be most useful when they returned to work at the end of the refresher course, red water appeared low on the list. Highest were advising farmers, carrying out injections, the restraint of animals, vaccines and buffalo management.

Again most (11) thought the course should have been longer, some to be able to absorb the information better, and practise more, while others wanted more information on other diseases and topics. In a ranking exercise on the methods they enjoyed most and felt best helped them to learn, treating cases brought to the clinic during the course, practicals and talks and discussions were highest with puppets and skits, field trips and slides lowest. Most felt the refresher course should be held between six months and a year after the beginners' course, and most said that Mangsir, Poush and Magh (mid-November to mid-February) was the best time to come for training. The trainees were largely happy with the accommodation and food.

The wide variety of comments at the end of the course – some wanted more information on horses, while others wanted less; some more on pigs, others less; and individuals wanting more on a wide variety of different topics – indicated that it is difficult to satisfy everyone with the same course, especially when they come from different parts of Nepal where livestock keeping and its problems may be very different. However, it was apparent that the majority were happy with the core content of the course.

FIELD VISITS

Introduction

The two sites for the field trips, Palpa and Lalitpur Districts, are located in the Western and Central Region respectively. Both areas are in the mid-hills with similar topography.

Baugha Pokhara Thok, the field site in Palpa, is about twelve kilometres from Tansen town, along a ridge away from the Palpa valley. Although it is close to town it is not as developed as some of the villages in the Palpa valley as it has no irrigated land. However, money comes into the village through the wages and pensions of men who are, or used to be, in the Indian army.

The field site in Lalitpur included the villages of Ikudol, Pyutar and Asrang. The three villages are fairly remote despite being less than fifty kilometres from Kathmandu, and near the district headquarters in Patan. To get there involves a one hour jeep ride to the road head at Tinpanebhanjang, and then between five and eight hours hard walking. The area is characterized by ridges and hills up to 8000 feet transected by river valleys 3500 feet below.

As the UMN Community Health Project has been active in the two areas for a number of years all four villages have Village Development Committees which have been selecting and sending farmers for VAHW training. Other project activities in the villages include agriculture and livestock, forestry, non-formal education, drinking water, rural industry and community primary healthcare. In Baugha Pokhara Thok, in addition to the CHP activities, the Government of Nepal has an agricultural service centre. The Government has also helped build a number of communal water systems, and is in the process of supplying electricity to the village. The Swiss Government has a programme in the area which includes water supply and community forestry. Despite all these activities, agriculture and especially livestock keeping are still largely traditional.

In contrast, the villages in Lalitpur have undergone many changes in livestock keeping and management over the past years. With the reduction of pastureage available since the establishment of community forestry plots and a voluntary ban on grazing, most animals are now stall-fed. As a result, there has been an increase in buffalo keeping and a decrease in cattle keeping. Buffalo give more milk and many people make khuwa (condensed milk) to sell in the Kathmandu valley. As little money is brought into the communities through wages, farmers are more dependent on the sale of livestock and livestock produce to provide cash income and are thus more interested in livestock improvement such as improved buffalo and goat cross-breeds.

Between 1981 and 1987, thirty-two farmers were sent from South Lalitpur for training as Village Animal Health Workers by AHITP. According to CDHP staff, twenty-four were still, in 1991, treating sick animals in their villages.

In Baugha Pokhara Thok, Palpa eight VAHWs have been trained by AHITP, and one by the government. Of the nine, seven were still active in 1991. One of the VAHWs, after working for several years, was employed by CHP as an extension worker, and another trained to replace him.

During the visits a number of rapid appraisal techniques were used including wealth ranking, mapping, diagramming and semi-structured interviews to learn about the area's social organization, agricultural and livestock practices, general and livestock-related problems, and how the village animal health workers were operating. However, during the shorter visit to Palpa (Baugha Pokhara Thok) it was decided to concentrate on the work that the VAHWs do and their relationships with the community and CHP.

All the villages are divided by the village development committees into wards of varying size, each having different sizes of farm and number of households. In Baugha Pokhara Thok, most aspects of the study were confined to people in Ward 1 of the nine wards of the village. On the Lalitpur visit, four wards were chosen for mapping in Ikudol. Farmers in Wards 1 and 2 were wealth ranked; in Ward 4 general problems of the ward were ranked, and a livestock calendar was constructed along with an analysis of the division of labour in livestock keeping. Interviews with villagers were conducted in Wards 1, 2, and 4. In Pyutar, the study team concentrated on Ward 3 which was mapped, and wealth ranked together with Ward 9, the adjacent ward. The livestock calendar and general problem ranking were both the work of farmers in Ward 3. Although four VAHWs were interviewed in Asrang only one farmer was interviewed from one of the Asrang wards.

While the primary intent of the field visits was to determine how well the VAHWs were working and how useful the farmers found their VAHW, the information gathered provides a social, economic and agricultural profile of the communities. Some of the findings are discussed in the sections to follow.

Palpa District

Most of the farms and dwellings in the village of Baugha Pokhara Thok are situated on the upland. All households have some land under crops but only one farmer has any irrigated rice land, and he has only 0.25 ropani (a sketch of the village drawn by one of the farmers is given in Figure 8). The main crops are millet, mustard and beans, with some farmers growing maize, buckwheat, black-grams, sugarcane and bananas. Most households keep some cattle and buffalo and goats, and many of the Magar people, who form the majority, and occupational castes keep pigs. Cattle and goats are taken out for grazing, but the buffalo are kept tethered and fodder is brought to them.

In the 1980s alone the number of houses nearly doubled (c.35 to 67), and the area for grazing decreased. There is now less uncultivated land, and some areas in the ward (and neighbouring wards) have been closed to grazing for community forestry projects. This has caused no major change in how people keep their cattle and buffalos, but, according to interviews with farmers, animal health has improved as a result of vaccination against haemorrhagic septicaemia and foot and mouth disease, and the work of VAHWs since 1987. There has, however, been a big increase in the number of people keeping pigs, and most are improved breeds. They are generally allowed to forage, but are fed some maize meal and rice husk.

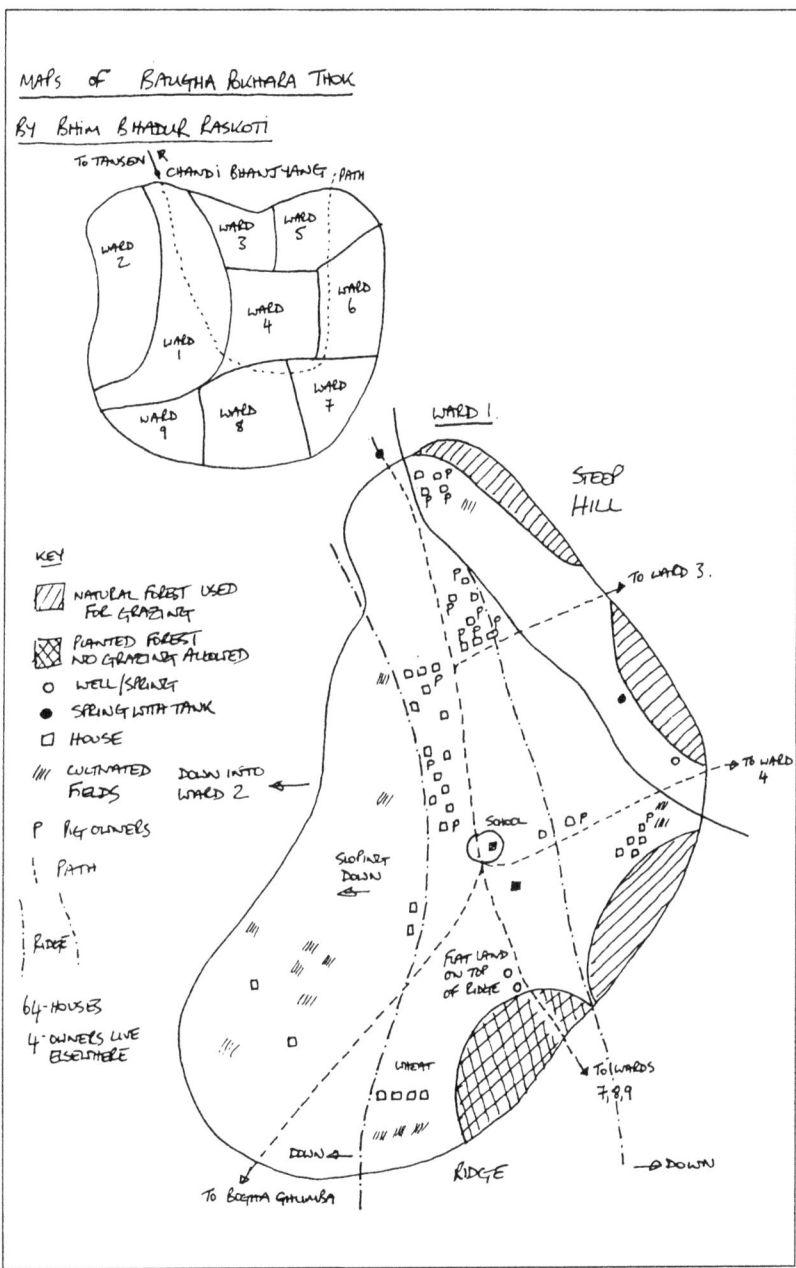

Figure 7: Map of Baugha Pokhara Thok

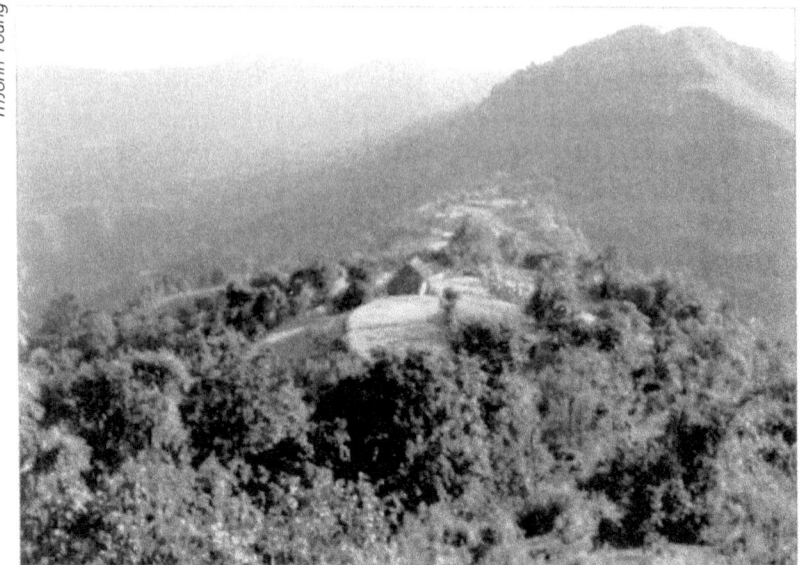

Baugha Pokhara Thok

A few Brahmins and Chettris sell ghee to Tansen, the nearby town, and to local consumers, but generally people consume most of the milk produced by their animals. On the other hand pigs are kept primarily to earn cash. Some people keep breeding pigs and sell piglets to other farmers. Some simply fatten the piglets and butchers come from Tansen to buy the fat pigs. It is very profitable because the meat sells for Rs.60 to 80 for 2.5 kilograms.

The sixty-seven households were organized into five wealth ranks by the former Pradhan Panch. There were seventeen households in the top rank, all with income from outside; some are, or were, in the Indian army and receive pensions, others have jobs. Some sell vegetables, ginger and molasses, and some have irrigated land in the Terai or Tansen and sell rice. Most have 40 to 50 ropani of upland. All have two or three buffalo, one or two cows, a pair of oxen, and a few goats and chickens. Magars and occupational castes have pigs, and sell piglets for Rs.400 or 500 at about five weeks old. These families can grow enough food for the whole year, and generally feed their entire maize crop to their animals.

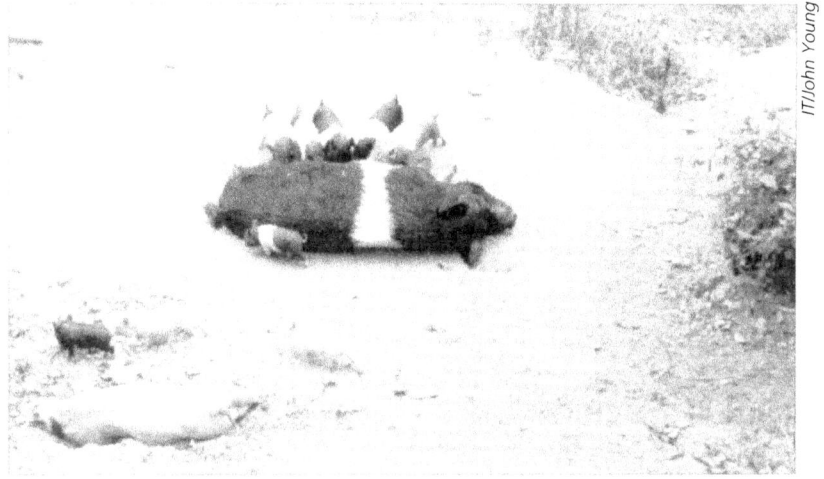

Pigs in Baugha Pokhara Thok

The ten households in Rank 2 receive less income from jobs and pensions and have about 25 to 30 ropani of upland. Some have to buy rice. They have roughly the same number and species of livestock as Rank 1 houses, but do not sell vegetables or other farm produce. Two are blacksmiths who make and repair sickles, sometimes in exchange for grain rather than for money.

Of the thirteen households in Rank 3, some are local blacksmiths and some are carpenters who go to other districts for four or five months each year to earn money. The others may have some external income, but many do not, and rely on their farms to provide food, which is generally enough for about ten or eleven months of the year. They have between 10 and 15 ropani of land, one or two buffalo and cattle, a pair of oxen, a few goats and some chickens.

The men from most of the seventeen households in Rank 4 work outside the district as carpenters building houses. At home they may have 10 to 15 ropani of upland but do not cultivate much because they buy food with the money they earn instead. They may have one or two buffalo and cattle, a couple of oxen, a pig and a few have goats and chickens. They may grow enough food for six to nine months.

The ten households in Rank 5 have four or five ropani of upland, but some have none and live on rich people's land as share croppers. Some have livestock of their own, and several look after livestock belonging to richer people, again for a share of the profits.

Many people now, especially in Rank 3, have less land than they had in 1980 as the land has been divided among the sons who tend to set up their own households rather than stay with their parents.

Slightly over half of the householders in the ward are Magar, but there are significant numbers of other castes as well. Magars form approximately half of all wealth ranks. Only ten per cent of the households are Brahmin, and they are all in the top three ranks, as are most of the Chetris except for two in the poorest rank. The occupational castes tend to fall in the lower ranks. Caste is significant in the village, not only in terms of wealth distribution, but in the consumption of meat (only Sarkis eat meat) and the rearing and butchering of livestock (pigs) regarded as unclean for Brahmins and Chetris. However, the VAHWs, all Magars except for one recently qualified Brahmin, treated the livestock of nearly all the castes in the village which suggests that caste was not an issue for either VAHWs or farmers.

In a ranking exercise where beans were used to weight general community concerns, lack of water for livestock was regarded as a pressing general problem. However, the lack of amenities such as health posts and electricity were ranked higher. A similar exercise focusing specifically on livestock problems showed that wealthier farmers regarded the lack of grass as a greater problem than lack of water, whereas poorer farmers felt the opposite. Both rich and poor ranked animal disease as the second problem. Interestingly, a livestock calendar constructed by a small group of farmers (Figure 8) showed that animal diseases are more prevalent just at the time when livestock are needed for ploughing.

Individuals also expressed a wide range of different problems when interviewed. Four out of five people mentioned the lack of enough labour and water as problems, three mentioned not enough

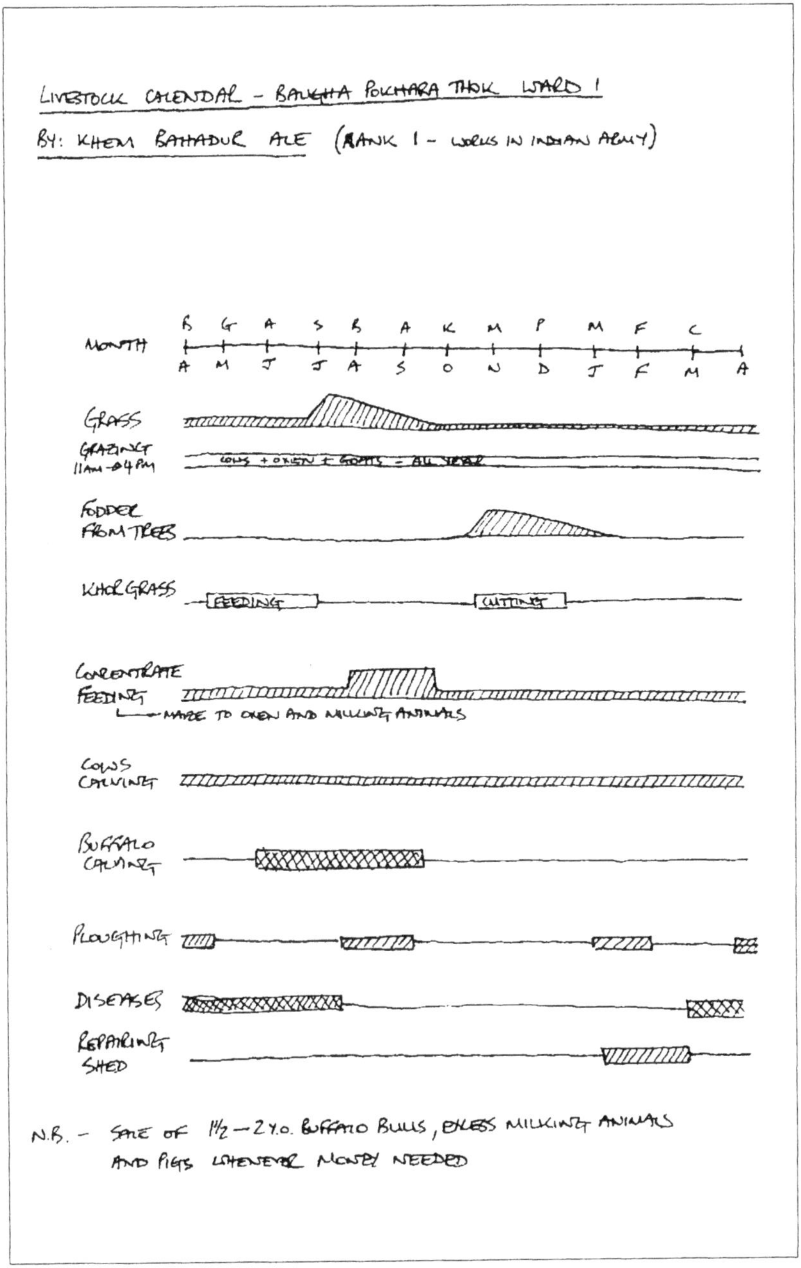

Figure 8: Livestock calendar in Baugha Pokhara Thok

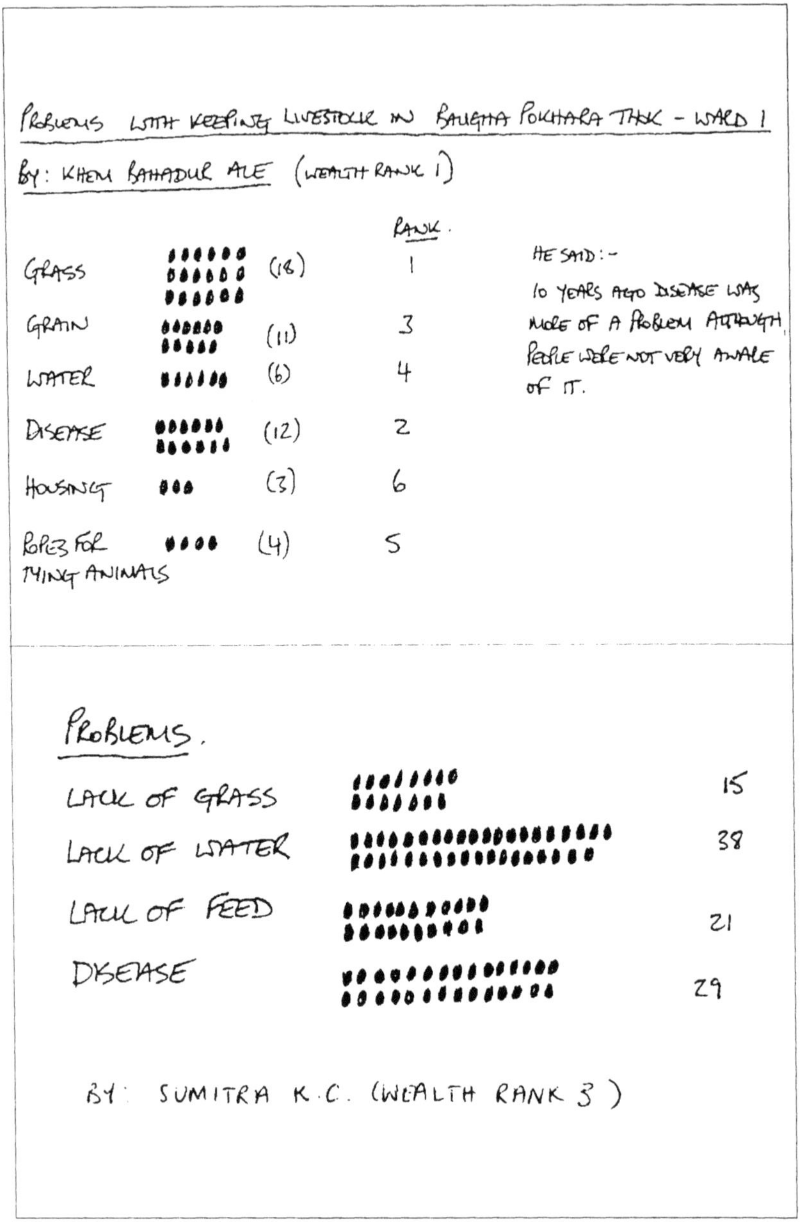

Problems with keeping livestock in Baugha Pokhara Thok - Ward 1
By: Khem Bahadur Ale (Wealth Rank 1)

		Rank	
Grass	●●●●●●●●●●●●●●●●●● (18)	1	He said :-
Grain	●●●●●●●●●●● (11)	3	10 years ago disease was
Water	●●●●●● (6)	4	more of a problem although
Disease	●●●●●●●●●●●● (12)	2	people were not very aware
Housing	●●● (3)	6	of it.
Ropes for tying animals	●●●● (4)	5	

Problems.

Lack of Grass	●●●●●●●●●●●●●●●	15
Lack of Water	●●●●●●●●●●●●●●●●●●●●●●●●●●●●●●●●●●●●●●	38
Lack of Feed	●●●●●●●●●●●●●●●●●●●●●	21
Disease	●●●●●●●●●●●●●●●●●●●●●●●●●●●●●	29

By: Sumitra K.C. (Wealth Rank 3)

Figure 9: Beanograms showing livestock problems in Baugha Pokhara Thok

grass, two the lack of feed for pigs. Poor housing, the lack of improved breeds, damage to crops from grazing, the poor grazing in the forests and disease were also mentioned.

VAHWs in Baugha Pokhara Thok
Prior to the training of the first VAHWs and when farmers were not aware of the veterinary hospital in Tansen, the village relied on the hankri. The owners of sick animals would touch the animal with some rice and take it to the Jhankri and describe the symptoms of the

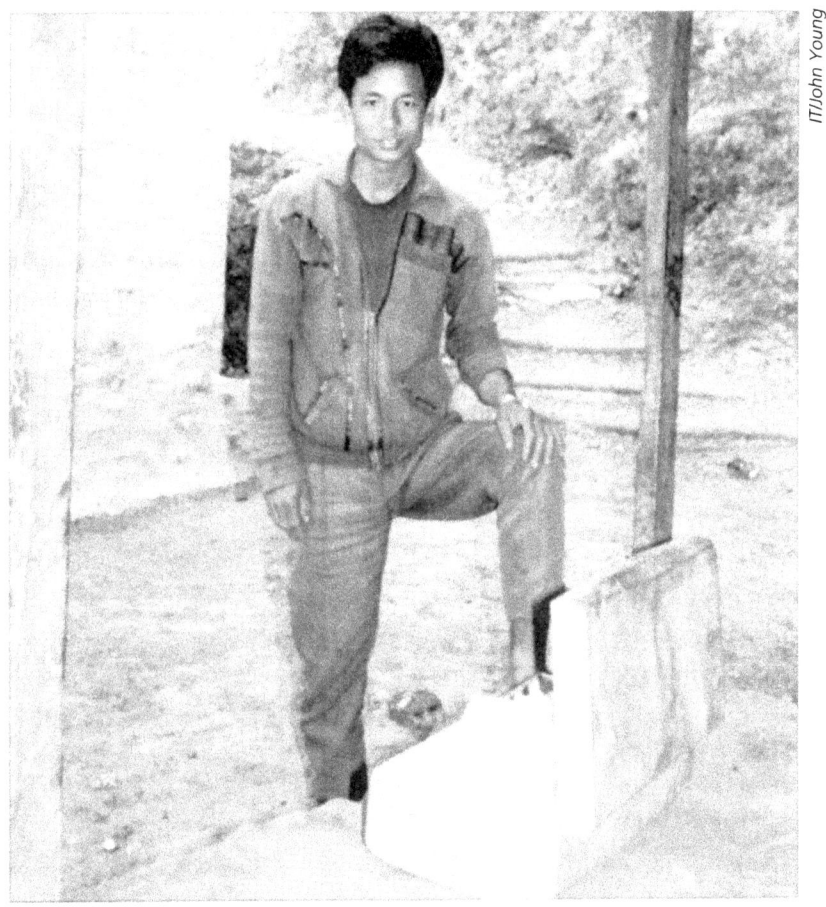

A VAHW with medicine box

disease. The Jhankri would then blow air on the rice. He never visited the sick animal, and prescribed no herbal medicine. In 1991, all the people interviewed were aware of the VAHWs working in their ward, most had used their VAHW, particularly for vaccinations against haemorrhagic septicaemia. They also were aware of alternatives; the veterinary hospital and the veterinary sub-centre in the adjoining VDC (one and a half hours walk from the village) where medicines are free of charge.

In Ward 1 an animal health committee has been established. The committee raised money to defray the costs of the medical kit for their recently-trained VAHW. It also fixes the fee schedule for the VAHW's services and receives fifty per cent of his fees. However, the VAHW serving in 1991 did not charge for his services and as the medicines were the property of the committee, he received no money for himself.

Of the nine VAHWs in the village six were interviewed, five of whom were still active in 1991. One gave up his VAHW work and returned his kit box to CHP: his son had left home leaving only himself and his wife to run the farm, and he was getting old. Another had left the area, but received further training at the government vet hospital, and was working at another village in the District. A VAHW from a neighbouring village was also interviewed.

All VAHWs had been selected for training by CHP staff, by committee meetings, or by influential members of the community, and most were or are engaged in other community work. One VAHW, a university student, felt he had been a poor choice as his studies kept him from the village, although he admitted being very busy when at home. Six of the seven interviewed had been sent by CHP. They had all been visited shortly after training by the project staff and at three monthly intervals since then. The six trained by AHITP had all received at least one follow up visit from AHITP staff. CHP had provided the medical kit for its trainees except in the case of the VAHW no longer practising. The VAHWs bought their medicines in Tansen, although the student VAHW prescribed medicines for the farmers to buy themselves.

The VAHWs treated a wide range of diseases, but they most commonly treated dystocia. They all treated parasites. The AHITP-trained VAHWs saw the benefit of their work in terms of serving the community and improving the health of their own livestock, not in terms of personal financial gains. The one non-AHITP-trained VAHW saw no benefit to his work.

The two main areas of concern expressed by the VAHWs were the lack of a reliable and accessible supply of medicine and equipment, and the lack of financial remuneration for their work. One VAHW expressed the need for another VAHW in his ward. They were generally happy with the training and support they received from AHITP and the project with a few suggestions for improvement: more training in specific areas, better accommodation, and more help with specific problems by the follow up staff.

South Lalitpur

The three villages of Ikudol, Pyutar and Asrang lie either side of a ridge which runs between the Khani Kola and Bagmati rivers. Farms in the three villages tend to be smaller than those in Baugha Pokhara Thok but with only marginally less livestock. Even among those farmers in Wealth Rank 1, the average size of farm was 18-20 ropanis with only one of 30 ropanis. However, more of the land is irrigated and is, therefore, more valuable: the yield from irrigated land can be 3-5 times greater than the yield from unirrigated land.

Ikudol is situated on the north side of the ridge above the Khani Kola river. Of the four wards visited in Ikudol, Ward 1 is on the top of the ridge, while Wards 2, 3, and 4 run down the side of the hill. Ward 1 has the poorest farms with only one farmer having irrigated land. Only three of the thirty-two households can grow enough grain to last for the whole year. The rest depend either on the sale of Khuwa, or the sale of livestock to buy grain, the poorest households depending on their wages as day labourers. Most households in the ward are Tamangs and goats' meat is consumed if it is available, especially around festival times. Few people in the ward have improved animals, but there are some cross-bred buffalo.

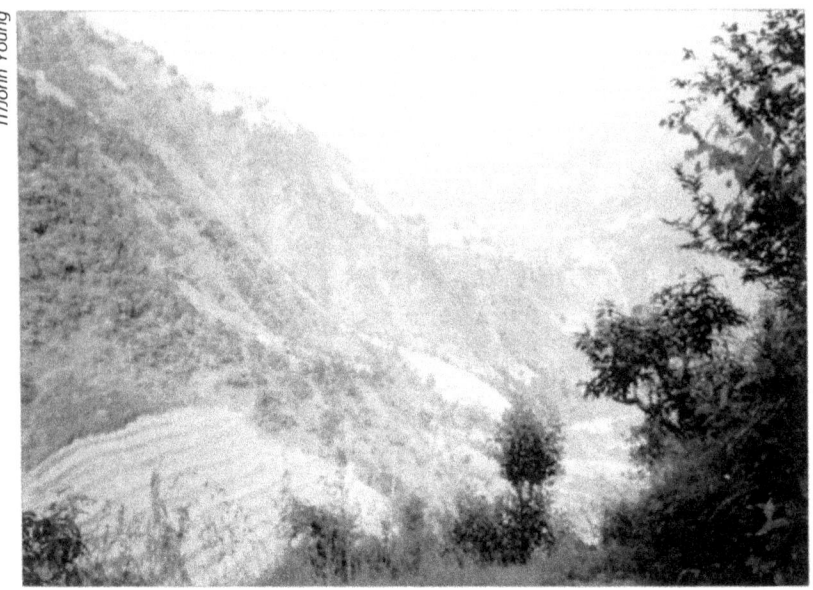

South Lalitpur

During the wealth ranking of Wards 1 and 2 it became apparent that different ethnic groups have settled in different parts of the village, with Tamangs at the top, and Brahmins and Chettris at the bottom where there is irrigated rice land. The mid-hill section is farmed mainly by Magars.

Farms below the ridge have buckwheat, mustard, wheat, maize and finger millet in the fields. The houses are surrounded by flowers, and there are vegetables including spinach, radishes and garlic. There have been no major changes in the crops grown and most are for home consumption. There are fewer cows and goats because of the restrictions on grazing. However, fodder trees provided by the CDHP agro-forestry programme have been planted for livestock feed. The buffalo have become the preferred livestock as they give more milk than cattle, particularly the improved breed. Also the Khuwa now produced from buffalo milk makes more money than ghee. The main problem in keeping livestock is the shortage of labour resulting from smaller families and from children attending school. There is now

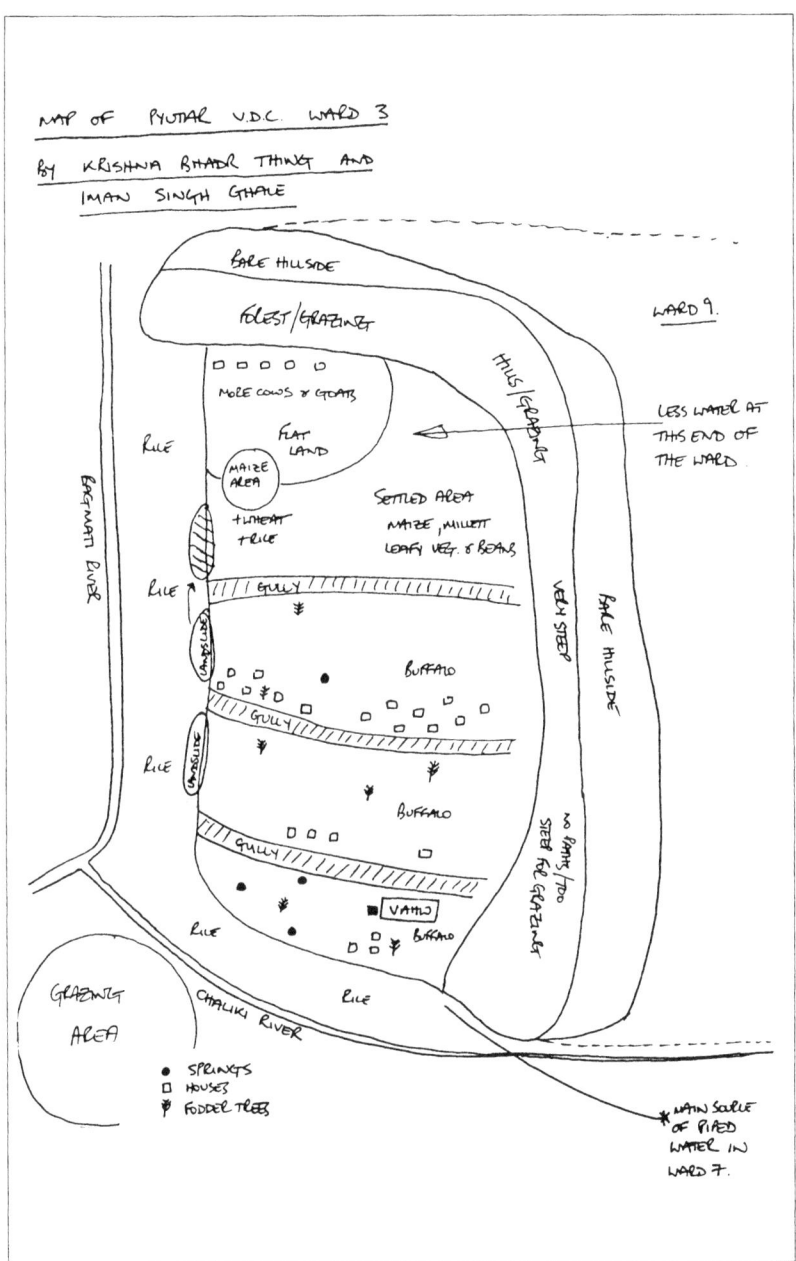

Figure 10: Map of Pyutar

piped water and everyone has their own tap, although drinking water is not available all year round.

General and livestock problem-ranking exercises were only undertaken in Ward 4. The two most urgent general problems were seen to be the lack of a grinding mill and the lack of electric light. Only two were livestock-related; a shortage of money for feed and the lack of buffalo bulls. In the livestock problem-ranking, diseases ranked highest, with lack of fodder and good housing being regarded as of least importance.

Pyutar is flatter, lower, and much more fertile than Ikudol. There are more people, the farms are closer together and a much wider range of crops is grown including rice, finger millet, various beans, pigeon peas, maize, vegetables, mustard, sesame, buckwheat, bananas and various fodder trees. There are more murrah and cross-bred buffalo and cross-bred cattle. It is ethnically more diverse, and closer to Hetauda, the headquarters of the District across the Bagmati – Makawanpur – than Patan the headquarters of Lalitpur District. As late as 1975, the whole hill behind the village was forested, and the area wetter. Vegetables grew better then, and there were more cattle and goats which were taken out grazing. On the other hand the Bagmati river was wider and less predictable, and now it is possible to cultivate more rice fields along its banks.

Pyutar's perceived general problems (Figure 11) were mostly different from those cited in Ikudol. Problems in common were deforestation, lack of drinking water, roads and schools. Along with lack of water, landslides and lack of seed and fertilizers ranked highest. Livestock problems in the two communities were the same, with diseases and access to treatment ranked first. Individuals more usually emphasized the lack of grass and the labour shortage as being more serious problems for livestock than disease, but in the ranking exercises, disease was always highest.

The progeny histories showed that loss from disease is a major problem especially for young animals: 20 per cent of buffalo calves die at less than six months old, 26 per cent of cattle die at less than one month old and 14 per cent of kids die before maturity.

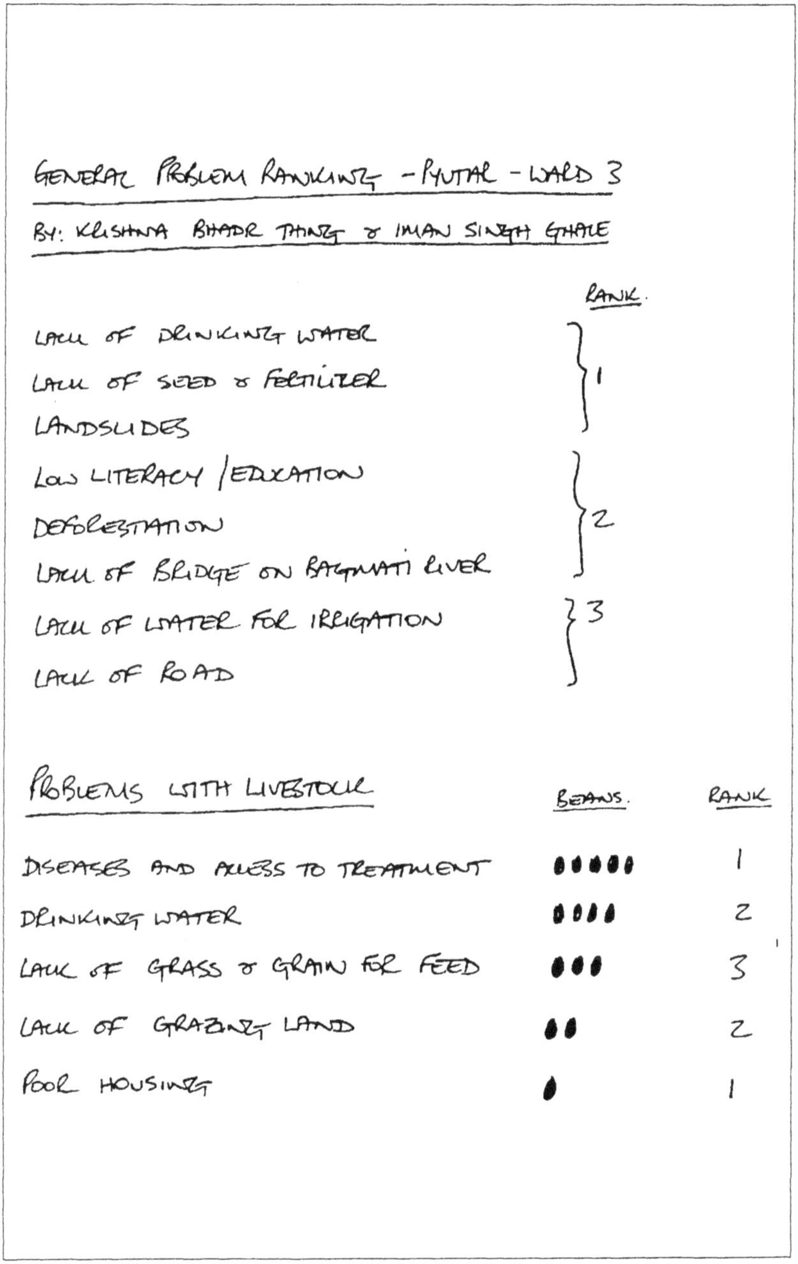

GENERAL PROBLEM RANKING - PYUTAR - WARD 3
BY: KRISHNA BHADR THING & IMAN SINGH GHALE

	RANK
LACK OF DRINKING WATER	
LACK OF SEED & FERTILIZER	1
LANDSLIDES	
LOW LITERACY / EDUCATION	
DEFORESTATION	2
LACK OF BRIDGE ON BAGMATI RIVER	
LACK OF WATER FOR IRRIGATION	3
LACK OF ROAD	

PROBLEMS WITH LIVESTOCK

	BEANS	RANK
DISEASES AND ACCESS TO TREATMENT	●●●●●	1
DRINKING WATER	●●●●	2
LACK OF GRASS & GRAIN FOR FEED	●●●	3
LACK OF GRAZING LAND	●●	2
POOR HOUSING	●	1

Figure 11: Beanograms of problems in Pyutar

VAHWs in South Lalitpur

When animals are sick many people in the villages continue to consult the Dhami-Jhankri before calling the village animal health worker, mainly because his services are free. Some people said the Dhami-Jhankri can treat loss of appetite, salivation and poor milk production, whereas other diseases need the medicines from the VAHW. The nearest veterinary sub-centre to Ikudol, Pyutar and Asrang VDCs is at Bhattedanda. It should be staffed by a JTA and a messenger, but it proved difficult to replace the last JTA when he left five months ago. Nevertheless the messenger who has worked there for many years keeps the sub-centre open and can provide medicines. Supervision of the staff at the centre is through visits by the supervisor (from Patan, the district headquarters) two or three times a year (although little technical advice was given on how to treat animals) and monthly staff meetings in Patan.

The centre had good supplies of herbal medicines including Pasupati Diarrhoea Powder, Pasupati Cough Powder and Pasupati Batissa. Supplies of carbon tetrachloride, Helatac, Hexathene, Piperazine, Nilverm, Terramycin and Penicillin were much poorer.

A maximum of fifty farmers used to visit the centre each month to ask for help, and the JTA would visit about twenty of them. The others just got medicine (if it was available). The medicine was free, but if the JTA visited the home there was a charge of Rs.50. Because the medicines are provided freely from the vet sub-centre, the JTA gained a lot of respect in the community. Only one of the farmers interviewed said that he went to the centre.

Many farmers felt that disease was now less of a problem in the areas as a result in part of the work of the VAHWs. Eleven of the fifteen interviewed were aware of the VAHWs and their work and most of that number had used them.

During the field trip eleven VAHWs were interviewed, six of whom treat many animals. Two were treating very few animals and three had stopped working as VAHWs altogether. Of the eight still active, one worked in Ikudol, four in Pyutar and three in Asrang. The VAHWs in Pyutar covered the greatest distances. Due to the low population density in the area, each VAHW serves only fifteen to thirty households. Despite that fact, some of the VAHWs reported a case load as high as eight to ten a month.

Selection of VAHWs for training was similar to the process in Baugha Pokhara Thok, but with the ward chairmen having a greater say in the final selection. All the VAHWs had received AHITP training and had been sent by CDHP who also provided the initial medicine kits. Three had taken government VAHW training in the past. All thought the AHITP training was good, and would like more, possibly in the field, combined with community mobilization work to make the community more aware of their services.

All liked the AHITP teaching methods, the practical approach and demonstrations with animals from the farm and clinic: one VAHW who had also experienced the one-month government course said that the only animals they saw in the whole period were two chickens!

Follow-up after training by CDHP staff had been frequent with help and advice given when requested. The CDHP staff who had themselves received VAHW training tended to be seen as points of referral and sources of medicine. Follow-up by AHITP staff appeared less consistent, with several of the VAHWs receiving no follow-up visits.

Although none of the VAHWs were able to show their records, the commonest diseases in the area were regarded to be liverfluke, internal and external parasites, foot and mouth disease, haemorrhagic septicaemia and anthrax. Much of the VAHWs work is in vaccination programmes, treatment of parasitic diseases and dystocias.

Some differences emerged in the population using the VAHWs. In Ikudol the VAHW serves rich farmers more than poor farmers, probably because they have more animals and the money to pay. In Pyutar the VAHW seems to serve rich and poor equally, but has served all the Brahmins and Chettris and not all of the other castes. The caste of the VAHW himself appeared to play no part in whether his services were used.

Of the two major problems for the VAHWs, access to medicine and non-payment by the farmers, lack of medicine caused them the most concern. Few of the VAHWs had much medicine in stock, and would need to go and get more before they could treat a sick animal. Many VAHWs have difficulty getting more medicines and the store keepers established by the CDHP do not maintain good stocks, thus the VAHWs are reluctant to buy from them.

The most active VAHWs have found their own independent source of medicines. An additional concern was the constantly changing names of the medicines which confused all the VAHWs.

Summary

While different social, economic and geographical factors make comparisons between the two field trips problematic, many of the issues and concerns of livestock and livestock production were shared by farmers in both areas. A couple of differences between the communities and their relationship with their VAHWs are notable, and have implications for AHITP in the future.

The VAHWs in South Lalitpur seem to regard themselves as independent workers with no great allegiance to the community, CDHP or AHITP although they look to CDHP staff to help with serious cases and the supply of medicines. This contrasted strongly with the prevailing attitude in Baugha Pokhara Thok where there was an Animal Health Committee who supported and worked actively with the VAHWs providing medicine kits and fixing fees. Although mention was made of the constraints this imposed on the VAHWs, several of them were also active in other types of work in the community and were themselves committee members.

In Baugha Pokhara Thok, everyone interviewed was aware of the existence of VAHWs in their area or ward, and now used them. This was not true in South Lalitpur, suggesting a need for more public relations work on the part of the project or the VAHWs themselves.

However, that the farmers valued the service provided by the VAHWs in both areas was more notable than any apparent differences between the two areas and there was general consensus that some diseases were less common since their arrival.

CONCLUSIONS

Although the animal health improvement training programme was established to train VAHWs for other UMN community development projects, by 1991 these projects had been more or less saturated, and AHITP was increasingly training VAHWs for other organizations. Of the 361 VAHWs trained since 1981, 180 were for other parts of the UMN, 141 for other international NGOs, 6 for a Nepali NGO, 11 for a government department and 23 for bilateral donor agencies. Now, to a much greater extent than in the past, AHITP is looking to find its place in the wider context of government livestock policy and to serve the training needs of NGOs and Nepali government departments.

No comparisons can be made between the content and quality of AHITP courses and other VAHW training courses available, but discussions with personnel from projects, other than CDP, who had sent farmers for AHITP training were favourable and requests for training increase steadily. Relations with most of the sending organizations have been good, and all the projects' staff interviewed were impressed with the training and the effectiveness of the trainees afterwards. Some partner projects would have liked AHITP to be able to offer a broader range of training for their staff and farmers. Even agencies who felt that the AHITP training was expensive, thought the quality of the course warranted the cost.

In 1992-3 the number of courses increased from 4 or 5 a year to 8 courses, and demand for training exceeded the capacity of the AHITP. For the first time since the experimental courses in 1981, a training course was held in the field in Jumla, using the facilities of the local veterinary hospital and agricultural centre.

The costs of the programme have been rising over the last few years. Since 1983, the cost of the project has increased steadily from about Rs.300,000 to about Rs.1 million in 1990-91. From 1988 to 1991, the cost of running the farm increased from Rs.80,000 to Rs.325,000 mainly because of salary increases.

In 1990-91, about seventy-five trainees attended two-week courses at the centre, bringing the cost to AHITP per trainee per course to about 14,000 rupees, but this does not include the cost of the medicine kit (Rs.2100). Including this cost, and the cost to the project of sending one staff member to the training, and the cost to the project of allocating staff time to support and follow-up the trainees (say 1 staff member for every 20 trainees, with an annual cost for that staff member of c. Rs.60,000) would bring the total cost to AHITP and the sending project per VAHW working in the field, to approximately Rs.19,000 (about £250).

In order to reduce the costs to AHITP, and with a view to establishing a more sustainable basis for the programme, AHITP charges projects about 25 per cent of the total cost to AHITP per trainee. Currently the fee is Rs.3500 (£50) per trainee per two week course, and this includes all training materials, including the trainee book and medicine book, and also one follow-up visit in the field by AHITP staff after training.

Although the farm is called the RDC farm, and is used to some extent by the other sections, it is of most use to, and is actually managed by the AHITP. The farm and clinic are operated out of one budget. Despite income generated from the sale of produce, from the clinic, and from accommodation and food for trainees attending, in 1990-91, there was a shortfall of Rs.325,000 – one third of the total cost of the programme. To cut costs, the farm has been reorganized and in 1992-3 the annual deficit was reduced to Rs.200,000. The more expensive trials such as the goat breeding trial have been finalized and greater emphasis has been put on productivity. In addition, extra income has been generated from charging all clients, including RDC, for the farm and clinic facilities and for the catering service.

The United Mission to Nepal has been going through a process of change. It is moving away from being mainly managed by expatriates, funded from abroad, and working independently of the government. It has been planning to increase the number of Nepali staff and to hand over the management of institutions including hospitals, schools, technical facilities and outreach programmes to the private sector (for example, the technical companies in Butwal) or the government (Gandaki Boarding School and Patan hospital). In 1992 AHITP replaced the expatriate veterinarian with a Nepali and employed a second JTA. The AHITP expatriate co-ordinator leaves in 1994 and is likely to be replaced by a senior Nepali staff person.

The Rural Development Department, of which the RDC is one project, plans to support local NGOs rather than run projects of its own, seconding expatriate staff directly to the NGOs. At the same time the UMN is looking for an increased local contribution to the costs of running the projects either from local communities through user charges or from charges to other organizations for services.

With the Rural Development Centre's move away from offering technical expertise to other projects to providing training services to community members and to other project staff, has come a strategic plan for 1992-7. The focus is hands-on, performance-based training, along similar lines to AHITP's training approach. It is keen to keep things simple, by offering a limited range of well-developed training courses, and to seek a greater impact by training trainers as well as community members. Special focus groups are women and occupational castes. It has been difficult to motivate projects to send women in the past, although there are examples of very effective female VAHWs.

With a view to the long term sustainability of its work, it is seeking to reduce costs, and to recover some (currently 25 per cent) of the costs from other organizations in Nepal. The RDC has been involved in an internal debate about the best structure and relationship with the UMN and the government.

Since the Nepali government's new Livestock Master Plan was formulated in 1991, Nepal's Ministry of Agriculture has undergone some significant changes. The Department of Livestock Services used to be one of four departments with its own regional and district level offices. A reorganization has resulted in one Agricultural Development Department with seven sections. In practice, this means that at Regional and District level matters concerning livestock development are under the direct responsibility of an agricultural officer, thus significantly reducing the livestock section's capacity to take decisions.

A key component of the plan was to increase the number of livestock extension workers, primarily self-employed VAHWs. With no detailed plan for the training of these VAHWs decided upon, it appeared that the Department of Livestock Services would need assistance from existing institutions such as AHITP to meet its training needs. However, with the DLS's loss of autonomy and government policy on livestock development and training VAHWs still unclear, AHITP cannot plan its future. One long-term option for RDC is that it should become an independent Nepali NGO, managed and staffed by Nepalis, and raising its own funds from international donors. It is apparent from the findings of the evaluation that AHITP has much to recommend it as an effective training facility.

The AHITP beginner and refresher courses are well-liked by the trainees, and are effective at passing on the knowledge and skills necessary for VAHWs to work successfully. The course content closely matches the most common and important diseases, and the short two-week duration enables AHITP to train more VAHWs than would be possible with a longer course. Nevertheless many of the trainees would like the courses to be longer, some want more information while others want more time to learn and practise. Trainees like the participative style of training, and especially the opportunity during the course to treat real sick animals, to practise handling livestock on the farm and to learn through talks and discussions. Most training takes place in the winter which trainees said was the best time.

The AHITP has developed an approach to the selection, support and follow-up of trainees which is very effective, but is dependent on good links with partner organizations for them to be implemented properly. Nevertheless more than 70 per cent are still working five years after training. Follow-up absorbs a lot of AHITP and partner staff time; medicine supplies are difficult to maintain, and even more difficult to ensure outside the control of a project; and some selection processes have resulted in the wrong trainees being chosen. Most of the VAHWs interviewed felt that the medicine kit developed by AHITP was good, and an important factor in establishing themselves as practitioners on their return home.

The AHITP farm and clinic provide a good venue for training, healthy animals and demonstrations of production systems and a steady supply of sick animals for trainees to treat through the veterinary clinic. However, as mentioned, the farm is very expensive to run and absorbs a third of the AHITP budget. Most of the cost is salaries for staff who spend part of their time looking after trials and demonstrations which provide little benefit to the programme. Some of the village surveys co-ordinated by AHITP have produced information which has been very useful to the development of training materials.

What has clearly emerged is the continuing need in Nepal for well-trained and dedicated VAHWs. As was apparent from the field visits, both in areas with a relatively high ratio of VAHWs to livestock, livestock health was a critical concern of the community. In a country of limited resources, a high density of livestock and unequal access to government veterinary facilities, VAHWs offer the best hope for an overall improvement in livestock health, a state of health on which many communities depend.

Appendix 1: Diseases treated by the Village Animal Health Workers

	No.	% of all work	% of disease
Vaccinations	2306	49	
HS vaccination	2267	48	
Other vaccination	39	1	
Internal parasites	1109	24	47
Liverfluke	656	14	28
Internal parasites	224	5	9
Small round worms	123	3	5
Large round worms	105	2	4
Tapeworm	1	<1	<1
External parasites	383	8	16
Mange	212	5	9
External parasites	95	2	4
Lice	74	2	3
Skin disease	2	<1	<1
Intestinal problem	430	9	18
Poultry diarrhoea	121	3	5
Digestive disorder	94	2	4
Diarrhoea	86	2	4
Anorexia	60	1	3
Bloat	36	1	2
Indigestion	15	<1	1
Poisoning	12	<1	1
Constipation	5	<1	<1
Bloody diarrhoea	1	<1	<1
Injuries and wounds	174	4	7
Wound	91	2	4
Abcess	69	1	3
Lameness	3	<1	<1
Eye injury	3	<1	<1
Broken leg	2	<1	<1
Broken horn	2	<1	<1
Caught	2	<1	<1
Broken bone	1	<1	<1
Maggots	1	<1	<1

Infections	110	2	5
Fever	39	1	2
Cough	30	1	1
Pneumonia	27	1	1
Mastitis	6	<1	<1
Eye infection	4	<1	<1
Black quarter	2	<1	<1
Foot and mouth	1	<1	<1
Haem. septicaemia	1	<1	<1
Urinary problems	42	1	2
Red water	36	1	2
Retained urine	6	<1	<1
Obstetrical problems	26	1	1
Retained placenta	9	<1	<1
Dystocia	9	<1	<1
Prolapsed uterus	5	<1	<1
Vaginal prolapse	1	<1	<1
Post partum fever	1	<1	<1
Anoestrus	1	<1	<1
Misc. diseases	25	1	1
Weakness	13	1	1
Allergy	5	<1	<1
Low temperature	3	<1	<1
Undiagnosed	3	<1	<1
Nervous disease	1	<1	<1
Routine procedures	75	2	3
Castration	60	1	3
Dehorning	11	<1	<1
Hoof trimming	2	<1	<1
Horn cutting	2	<1	<1
Total treatments	4680		
Total (not vacc.)	2374		

Source: AHITP follow-up reports. (NB – this represents only those cases for which records are available, and gives an indication of the relative numbers of different diseases/conditions treated not the total amount of cases treated by all the VAHWs since the project began.)

Appendix 2: Beginners' course contents

- Sick animal examination
  Question asking and examination techniques
  Record keeping
  Use of the thermometer
- Restraint of animals
  With ropes
  Casting
  Construction and use of a crate
- Care of sick animals (feed, housing)
- Tour of the farm facilities and demonstrations
  Silage making, fodder trees, appropriate housing and feeding systems
- Internal parasitism (treatment and prevention)
  Liverfluke, large round worms, small worms (nematodes)
- External parasitism (treatment and prevention)
  Fleas, lice, ticks, nasal leeches, mange, ringworm
- Proper use of medication
  Precautions when handling toxic medicines
  How to measure dosages of powders and liquids
  Use of a syringe and preparation of sterile injections
- What is fever and how to treat it
- Castration using a burdizzo
- Digestive diseases
  Anorexia, diarrhoea, constipation, poisoning, bloat
- Contagious/infectious diseases
  Haemorrhagic septicemia, pneumonia, foot and mouth disease, wounds, abscesses, eye infections
- Calving problems
  Dystocia, retained placenta, prolapsed uterus
- Fractures and broken horns
- Book-keeping (how to charge, keep financial records, buy medicine)
- How to teach farmers
- What to expect during follow-up field visits from AHITP and project staff
- Field trips to see raising of pure bred 'improved' breeds and the local veterinary district hospital

Appendix 3: Refresher course contents

- Buffalo husbandry and management
- Goat husbandry and management
- Fodder trees, hay making, stall feeding and nutrition
- Water buffalo breeding, heat detection and infertility problems
- Poultry and swine husbandry (includes vaccination and boar castration)
- Equine diseases:
  colic, parasitism, lameness
- Infectious diseases:
  bloody urine (red water), rabies, anthrax, black quarter
- Proper use of antibiotics and vaccines
- Allergic reactions
- Sub-normal temperatures and milk fever
- Pig diseases:
  hog cholera, diarrhoea, worms, mange, agalactia
- Hand-rearing of orphans
- Tapeworms and gid
- Mastitis and milking techniques
- Hoof trimming

Appendix 4: The AHITP recommended medicine kit

Medicine		Use	Quantity
Himalayan batissa		Anorexia	1kg
Timpol		Bloat	1kg
Neblon		Diarrhoea	1kg
Sodium thiosulphate		Poisoning	
Magnesium sulphate		Constipation	
Sulphur		Mange	
Hexathene		Liverfluke	2kg
Panacur		Intestinal worms	
Proc. penicillin:	2 mil IU	Injectable antibiotic	6 vials
	4 mil IU	Injectable antibiotic	12 vials
Penidur	2.4 mil IU	Injectable antibiotic	9 vials
	600,000 IU	Injectable antibiotic	6 vials
Terramycin 50mg/ml 30ml		Injectable antibiotic	5 vials
Vitamin B	30ml	Anorexia, anaemia	5 vials
Cural	30ml	Poisoning/allergy	
Piperazine tablets		Large worms	30
Sulphadimidene tablets		Diarrhoea/obstetrical	50
Himax tubes		Maggots/insects	5
Terramycin eye tubes		Conjunctivitis	2
Malathion 5% powder		Fleas/lice	1kg
Savlon		Antiseptic	0.3 l
Tetmosol soap			1
Cotton wool 150 g			1

Equipment

Stomach tube for goat		1
Stomach tube for cow		1
Syringe	10ml	5
Syringe	20ml	2
Needles	16g	2
	18g	2
	20g	2
Plastic roll		0.5kg
Turpentine oil		0.1 l
Iodene tincture oil		0.1 l
Tin box		
Padlock		

www.ingramcontent.com/pod-product-compliance
Ingram Content Group UK Ltd.
Pitfield, Milton Keynes, MK11 3LW, UK
UKHW021831140426
5217IPUK00021B/1377